© **Copyright 2**

By Pauline PATRY – SAS[...] [rig]hts reserved. No part of this publi[cation] [may be reproduced, stored] in a retrieval system, or transmi[tted in any form or by any mea]ns, including photocopying, re[cording, or other electronic] or mechanical methods. All rights reserved. This book is protected by copyright law.

The opinions and the information contained in this book are under no circumstances a substitute for medical advice or treatment. First and foremost, you must follow a doctor's advice. The author rejects all responsibility which might arise out of the use of this work. The author is not responsible for what the reader does with this information, under any circumstances.

The contents of this book is for informational purposes only and are meant to be discussed with your physician or other appropriate healthcare professional. Never disregard medical advice dispensed by your doctor or other qualified healthcare professional. Always seek the opinion of a physician with any question you may have regarding a medical condition as well as before undertaking any actions which might affect your health. The information in this book is not intended as a substitute for medical advice. It is important to speak to your doctor about what is claimed in this book before taking any action. Because each case and each person is unique, we cannot guarantee any result with this book.

Overcoming Burnout

Complete Guide to Burnout Recovery

Burnout Prevention & Treatment

How to Recover from Job Stress & Burnout

Pauline PATRY

Table of Contents

Table Of Contents 3
Introduction 4
Chpt 1: 5 Risk Factors For Burnout 8
Chpt 2: Stages Of Burnout 12
Chpt 3: 10 Signs Of Burnout 15
Chpt 4: Tips To Stop Burnout Before It Starts 18
Chpt 5: Burnout Relief Strategies 21
Chpt 6: Prevent Burnout With Simple Strategies From Psychologists ... 24
Chpt 7: The Aftermath Of Burnout: How To Rejuvenate Yourself 27
Chpt 8: Understanding Burnout Associated With The Workplace 29
Chpt 9: Are You Suffering From Workplace Burnout? 32
Chpt 10: Passive Income: Prevent Burnout And Enrich Your Business. 38
Chpt 11: Why You Must Stress Less 48
Chpt 12: How To Manage Normal Stress 53
Chpt 13: Meditation 59
Chpt 14: 3 Top Ways To Reduce Everyday Stress 67
Chpt 15: How To Manage Anxiety And Panic Attacks 69
Chpt 16: How To Calm Yourself Down In Stressful Situations 71
Chpt 17: How To Use The 80/20 Principle To Reduce Stress 74
Bonus Chapter 76
Final Words 84
Your Gift: Free Ebook About Alkaline Foods 85
Your Feedback On This Ebook 87

Introduction

It is kind of obvious once you have hit burnout, the exhaustion, lack of motivation, poor efficacy, and overwhelming doubts of whether you should even be at your job are hard to miss. But, if you are not there yet, perhaps the symptoms aren't as obvious.

So what is burnout? Burnout is the result of too much stress either from your job, a life situation, or even your personality. In the simplest of terms, burnout is absolute exhaustion, physical, mental, and emotional.

It is a combination of symptoms that cause you to be much less effective at work, less happy at home, and if left unchecked could cause your serious health complications. Burnout can leave you anxious, depressed, unmotivated, and ineffective. The list of symptoms can be vague and sound like just life, but life isn't supposed to feel like Burnout.

The usual signs of burnout are constant feelings of helplessness, irritability, anxiety attacks, weight loss or weight gain and insomnia. Symptoms of burnout can affect the emotional, mental and physical well- being of a person. Burnout is a state of exhaustion. This is typically caused by prolonged and excessive stress. It is experienced when someone feels overwhelmed by the everyday demands of work and that person is unable to meet the demands because of certain reasons.

Burnout is very common among healthcare workers most especially to medical assistants or MAs. Possibly, it can be due to the constant pressure, long hours of work and the demanding workloads that come along with their everyday routine.

Burnout may have a negative effect on the person's relationships and engagements at home and at work. Prolonged stress can reduce one's productivity and later. Moreover, burnout can make a person feel cynical, restless, sarcastic and resentful. It can also cause one's body to be vulnerable to various illnesses such as common colds and flu. Burnout must be managed effectively before it gets worse.

Work Burnout is Dangerous to your Health!

If you are a business owner or an employee, the holidays can be overly busy times. You feel the responsibility to your customers and clients. Added personal responsibilities for the extra time needed to get gifts, attend social events can make you feel like you are burning the candle at both ends. Where is the time going to come from? This added pressure can bring you to the point of burnout.

Work burnout is a common occurrence among the best and most responsible workers in all fields. It happens most frequently if you love your job and what you do. You have high standards for yourself;

Perhaps you are a bit of a perfectionist or an idealist. You want to provide the best service; go over and beyond what is expected to give service to others.

Burnout can sneak up on you. You may not even realize that it is work that is causing your symptoms, and think that you are feeling stress from other areas in your life. In fact, whether the cause is work or other stress, your symptoms can overlap. Burnout can even seem like depression, and often doctors will misdiagnose and mistreat work burnout. That is why it's important for you to be aware of the symptoms. If you are dealing with another stressor in your life, and you don't feel better, you can start feeling frightened and powerless about getting better.

With work burnout, as you get busier and busier trying to get more accomplished, it becomes almost like the syndrome of a frog in slowly increasing warm water getting boiled to death. You don't even notice until it's too late.

Stress or Burnout - What is the Difference?

Stress and burnout are often seen as the same thing. But they are not the same.

Stress happens to everyone every single day! Each person experiences and copes with stress very differently. What is stressful to you may not be to me... and vice versa! And how you react to stress and cope with it will be very different to the way I do.

Most people see burnout as only happening to high-powered, overworked business executives. But the reality is, burnout can happen to almost anyone – it is not reserved to a select group of people in a select area of work!

Burnout can occur in caregivers (for example, someone who's sole caregiver for a chronically or seriously ill person over a long period of time e.g. with Alzheimer's disease), executives, stay at home mums or dads with several young children, health care workers (e.g. doctors, psychologists, nurses, vets)... to name a few. In other words... it can happen to anyone doing too many tasking things over a long period of time.

So... what is burnout? And what is the difference between burnout and stress?

Well... according to Wikipedia, "burnout is a psychological term for the experience of long-term exhaustion and diminished interest."

And according to Wikipedia, "stress is the condition that results when person-environment transactions lead the individual to perceive a discrepancy, whether real or not, between the demands of the situation and the resources of the person's biological, psychological or social systems."

There is a huge difference between burnout and stress. Stress is a normal part of daily living... every single person experiences some degree of stress in their lives each day. Burnout, on the other hand, may be the result of unrelenting stress, but it isn't the same as too much stress.

Stress is an overload of pressure that demands too much of you both physically and psychologically. People experiencing stress can usually see that they will feel better when they can get everything under control.

Burnout, on the other hand, is prolonged stress and pressure. It is emotional and physical exhaustion caused by excessive and prolonged stress. It results in feeling empty, totally exhausted, very overwhelmed, and devoid of motivation.

Burnout reduces your productivity and saps your energy. It may leave you feeling increasingly helpless, hopeless, powerless, often cynical and resentful. People experiencing burnout very seldom see there is any likelihood of feeling better. They begin to lose interest and motivation that led them to take on the roles and responsibilities in the first place e.g. being a caregiver. The unhappiness of burnout causes can eventually threaten your job, your relationships and your health.

Another major difference between stress and burnout is: usually you are aware you are under a lot of stress, but you usually don't notice burnout when it happens. The symptoms of burnout including total exhaustion, feelings of detachment, hopelessness, often take months to appear.

It is not uncommon for someone else to point out you may be experiencing burnout... many people with burnout don't see it in themselves. More often than not, work colleagues, family members, partners, friends, or doctors will see the signs of burnout long before the person sees it in him or herself.

If the signs are recognized in time... burnout can be prevented or alleviated. I'm not saying for one moment that everyone will experience burnout... far from it! But burnout does exist... it is real and its effects can be devastating if not recognized and dealt with effectively.

Chapter 1
5 Risk Factors for Burnout

A risk factor is a variable whose presence increases your risk for problems. For example, you are at higher risk of disease if several risk factors are present. This chapter discusses the risk factors for experiencing burnout.

Burnout is a psychological term for a set of characteristics usually centering around stress and exhaustion, especially in one's career. If you are feeling apathetic, mentally fatigued, having difficulty concentrating or difficulty caring, these could be emotional warning signs of burnout. If you find yourself avoiding work, neglecting your responsibilities, being accident prone and disregarding your appearance,

you may be experiencing behavioral signs. If you suffer from insomnia, headaches, fatigue or increased worrying about your health, these may be physical signs of burnout.

Paying attention to these warning signs is vital to avoiding burnout. It is possible to have some emotional, behavioral and physical signs present and you may or may not have associated these signs as signs of burnout. Here are five risk factors for burnout. Are these risk factors present in your life?

Your Perception of Stress

In my stress management workshops, I have an exercise where I ask participants to list the things that cause them stress and then as a group, we list them on chart paper. Inevitably, there are some people who will say that they are not stressed by some of the things listed. For example, some people find traveling stressful while others do not. Some people find deadlines stressful while others see it as a motivator. Albert Ellis, a prominent psychotherapist in the field of cognitive therapy, discovered that this is due to our perception of stress. He pointed out that our underlying beliefs and self-talk contribute a great deal to our stress and that changing these underlying beliefs and self-talk are key to reducing stress. If you perceive your current situation to be stressful, you will experience more stress than someone in the same situation who perceives it as manageable. No two people in the same situation view the situation in the same way and this is how your perception of stress is a risk factor for burnout.

Stress at Home

It is difficult to have stress at home and act like nothing is wrong when you get to work. Even if you do not share your troubles with your co-workers, chances are you have a shorter fuse than if you had very little stress at home. You may come into work tired, take longer to focus on work, think about how much time is left before you can leave for the day or the weekend. Whatever is going on at home stays in the back of your mind during your time at work and reduces your ability to give 100% of your attention to work. As a result, your performance can suffer over time.

Environmental Stress

Stress can come from the environment you live in as well. We do not often notice environmental stress because we tolerate them for the most part. Environmental stress can come from traffic, weather, neighbors, crime level, noise, the economy, etc. Sometimes environmental stress can be lessened. For example, if you have a long commute to and from work, you can find a way to change your work hours, work from home, change jobs, or move. Most of the time, we just put up with this form of stress and cease to think about it. The problem with this is that any stress, whether you have found a way to tolerate it or not, is using your body's resources to keep you going despite the stress. That means that you have less resources to handle other stress in your life.

Work Stress

All jobs have some level of stress associated with them and some jobs have more stress than others. But chronic stress that is above and beyond what is considered a given in the profession can lead to burnout. If, in addition to the regular stress associated with your job, you are dealing with a boss with poor leadership skills or the negative effects of low morale amongst your co-workers (i.e. complaining, gossiping), this can lead to increased stress and decreased work performance.

Not Practicing Stress Management

This is a major risk factor for burnout. Stress is everywhere and you can only tolerate so much before succumbing to the effects of burnout. Practicing stress management on a regular basis is vital to counteract the effects of stress. Stress uses up your body's resources, including your physical, mental and emotional stamina. Just like a car needs gas to keep going, your body needs replenishment to keep going. That replenishment is stress management. You would not expect your body to continue to function at peak performance if you did not eat every day. Yet many people expect their minds, bodies, and emotions to function at peak performance without stress management. Eventually, your tank hits empty and the road to full can be a long one. Regular stress management practice can avoid this and keep you functioning at peak performance on a regular basis.

What is your risk factor for burnout? Rate your perception of stress on a scale of 1 to 5 where 1 is very little stress and 5 is more stress than you can handle. Rate your stress at home on a scale of 1 to 5 where 1 is very little stress and 5 is more stress than you can handle. Rate your environmental stress on a scale of 1 to 5 where 1 is very little stress and 5 is more stress than you can handle. Rate your work stress on a scale of 1 to 5 where 1 is very little stress and 5 is more stress than you can handle. How often do you practice stress management? Rate yourself from 1 to 5 where 1 is every day and 5 is not very often.

If you scored below 10, your risk of burnout is low. Congratulations.

If you scored 10-15, you are at risk of burnout. As I mention in my book, The Art of Loving Life, one of the 3 steps to controlling stress is to remove what is causing you stress or reduce your stress with one of the clinically proven, time-tested techniques described.

If you scored above 15, you probably do not need me to tell you that you are burned out. Take immediate steps to deal with your stress. A competent therapist or coach who is skilled at stress management can help you.

Chapter 2
Stages of Burnout

The experience of burnout is not an overnight event. Burnout is something that develops over time because we fail to recognize the warning signs and do something about them. We recognize that warning lights and strange sounds coming from our car means it is time to find out what is wrong and fix it. But we often ignore the warning signs coming from our bodies. I will talk about the five stages of burnout so that you can better recognize the warning signs and have the opportunity to do something about them before the effects of burnout take over your body, mind, and life.

There are five stages of burnout. There are no set rules on how you will progress from one stage to another. How long you stay in each stage is dependent on your particular situation. You may stay in a particular stage for years and never advance to the next stage. You may make adjustments in your life that will bring you to a lower stage of burnout or out of burnout completely. No matter what stage you find yourself in, it is never too late to make adjustments that can improve your life.

Honeymoon Stage

This is the stage you find yourself in when you start a new job or a new project. Regardless of what the new event is, you dive in wholeheartedly. You do not mind the long hours, the extra demands on your attention and energy or the learning curve required to be successful in this new challenge. You are happy and you love everything about this new opportunity even if it is stressful. The downside of this stage is that you are going along completely unaware of the toll it takes on your mind, emotions, and body to maintain this high level of productivity. You could be close to running on empty and not even know it.

Speed Bump

After a while, you start to notice that you are not functioning like you used to. Maybe you are a little tired. Maybe you notice that you are making mistakes here and there. You begin to work even harder to maintain the same level of productivity you started off with. Part of you recognizes that you need a break. However, if you do not take that break, you will start to see some of the signs of burnout I talked about in my last article. The job, the project, the event will not be as exciting as it used to be and you may not be as enthusiastic as you used to be about working on it. When you do work on it, you may find that you are not as productive or effective as you used to be. You may have difficulty shutting your mind off. Whereas in the honeymoon stage, you did not mind thinking about it all the time but now it is negatively affecting your ability to sleep or leave it behind to have fun. This can lead to compensating behaviors such as overeating, drinking, or shopping to "reward" yourself for working so hard.

Chronic Stress Stage

This is the stage where you no longer deny that something is happening to you. You may or may not connect your symptoms to the new job, project or event, but you no longer deny that you need help managing your symptoms. You may see a doctor for help sleeping or for headaches or stomach problems. Your problems are probably not limited to the physical realm either. You may be feeling constantly irritated, worried, have difficulty concentrating and feel overwhelmed. This is a critical stage. This is the stage where most people seek stress management in the form of a vacation, a new job, a new project, and/or medication. The danger is in finding yourself in the honeymoon stage again only to progress back to this stage. This cycling around the honeymoon stage, the speed bump, the chronic stress stage and back again can be avoided with regular stress management practice. As mentioned in The Art of Loving Life, awareness is the key to managing stress. Increasing your awareness of the stages of burnout and its particular effects on you can save you from having to cycle through these stages again and again. It can certainly save you from progressing to the next stage.

Crisis Stage

At this stage, you become a walking time bomb. The symptoms of the chronic stress stage have exacerbated but your efforts to cope are ineffective. You may get fired, become hospitalized, experience serious relationship problems or cause significant problems for others. You may find yourself worrying about worst case scenarios which can lead to extreme thoughts, such as running away, suicide, bankruptcy, and other fantasies of escaping from your life.

Exhaustion Stage

In this burnout stage, exhaustion implies that your mind and body's resources have been completely used up. You have been hospitalized for a major illness, suicide attempt or alcohol/drug addiction or in jail due to a distorted attempt to escape your situation. Recovery from this stage is a long process. At this stage, it takes more than stress management to recover but recovery is possible with professional help.

Recovery is actually possible at any stage. Regular stress management can help you maintain your honeymoon stage level of productivity and reduce the likelihood of your reaching the speed bump stage or beyond. If you recognize that you are at the chronic stress or exhaustion stage, please seek professional help. Incorporating stress management, even at these stages is helpful and can complement other forms of professional help but stress management alone is not enough.

Chapter 3
10 Signs of Burnout

Let's just face it, we are all overworked and underpaid. We want to take a vacation but don't for fear of falling too far behind. We want to go to the doctors but, our health insurance plan only covers one visit a year. Sound familiar? If so, you might just be experiencing job burnout! Take a peek at the following ten signs of burnout. Having only a few means you are getting close, having more than a few means you need a vacation!

Job Burnout Sign #1: Chronic Fatigue

If you are overtired and taking several doses of ibuprofen each day hoping that headache will go away, you are probably experiencing chronic fatigue. This is a symptom many workaholics experience.

Job Burnout Sign #2: Anger, Irritability

Have you ever been so angry with a customer that you wish you could just tell them how you really feel? Or what about telling your boss how you really feel? Well, most people call that anger or irritability. While these are also symptoms many workaholics experience, it could also be a sign you need a new job!

Job Burnout Sign #3: Self-Criticism

We all have those days where no matter what we do, we feel like we just can't get it right. Good news for those of you who feel that way on a day-to-day basis! Chances are you are delirious from being overtired when you feel like what you did isn't good enough, even though it is probably great and fussing with it, even more, may just ruin it! Leave a good thing alone!

Job Burnout Sign #4: Negativity

If you have ever had a moment where you hate the world, or your boss, or your in-laws, you may be experiencing negativity. This is also a symptom many workaholics experience.

Job Burnout Sign #5: Weight Loss or Weight Gain

Have you ever purchased a new pair of work pants and kept them in your closet until your big presentation, except, when you go to put them on for that presentation, you can't seem to button them? Or have you gone to work with your shirt fitting better than your sweatshirt and dress pants fitting more comfortably than your sweats? Well, it may have something to do with that all coffee and donut diet or starvation because of stress diet!

Job Burnout Sign #6: Sleeplessness

This one is always fun! Tossing and turning because you can't seem to fall asleep than when you do fall asleep all you do is dream about work, which of course, wakes you up anyway because I do believe that is categorized as a nightmare!

Job Burnout Sign #7: Depression

Are you feeling sad, mopey or just plain miserable? Are you replacing water for wine at the dinner table? Started smoking cigarettes? Rather stay in the house than get outside and breathe in the fresh air? Well, you could be depressed.

Job Burnout Sign #8: Feelings of Helplessness

This is a great one! Usually goes hand in hand with depression. Curing one would cure them both, so, go on a vacation or start looking for a new job!

Job Burnout Sign #9: Increased Degree of Risk Taking

This is that lovely feeling of "I just don't care" because the consequence may actually be the reward. If you don't care about getting fired because you have been trying to get fired, you may be working too much, and at the wrong job!

Job Burnout Sign #10: You Think You Are Burnt-out

This is the most obvious symptom! If you are sitting in a chair with your hand to your forehead saying, "I am just burnt-out," you are probably right!

Chapter 4
Tips to Stop Burnout Before it Starts

People suffering from burnout may experience a number of physical and emotional problems, including exhaustion, anxiety, and depression. If you're burned out but you won't change your lifestyle in substantial ways, health problems as severe as heart attacks or strokes may be in your future.

You should learn to recognize the distinctive warning signs of burnout so that you can take steps to prevent serious health problems from developing. It may be that only simple changes are needed in your life to completely sidestep burnout.

You can prevent burnout by following these tips:

1. Evaluate Your Workload. Many people take on workloads that are far too heavy, forgetting that they won't have enough time in the day to complete all the tasks. Burnout will result if you constantly tackle your workload at full speed without taking any breaks. If you want to change your approach to work, you have two choices:

• First, you can learn how to work more efficiently with the help of time management strategies. The idea is to do more work in less time.

• Second, you can eliminate unnecessary tasks from your schedule. You may not believe this can be done if you're a true workaholic, but you'll have to find a way if you want to preserve your health and happiness.

2. Don't Overwork. If you have a good mind-body connection, you'll know when you're reaching your exhaustion limit. When you reach this point, you must stop working and initiate some change. For some people, spending the day relaxing at home is enough; others may want to take a short vacation or spend the day in a favorite spot. The point of this is to get away from those things that cause you the most stress. If your major sources of stress are cell phones and computers, leave them behind for a day!

3.   Welcome, Change. If burnout is occurring over and over again in your life, then it's time you commit to a major life change.

For example, your job may be a source of constant burnout no matter what you do to steer clear of it. If this is the case, you may need to find a job that you're better suited to.

4.   Schedule Regular Breaks. Employee breaks are now mandatory, and there's a good reason for that. Workers need to take time out to regroup and refresh themselves. On your break, you can probably take a short walk, work on a Sudoku puzzle, or find some other way to alleviate your stress, even if just for a few minutes.

5.   Don't Hesitate to Ask For Help. People often get so wrapped up in their problems that they fail to seek help from others - even when this help may be exactly what is needed to remove stress. It's important for you to have someone in your life you can go to for advice or just for a listening ear, whether it is your partner, a friend, or a therapist.

6.   Just Say No. Saying yes to everything and being accommodating are two very different approaches to life. If you're a yes-person, you're making yourself vulnerable to others who might take advantage of you. Sometimes the best thing you can do is just say no. Saying yes all the time can cause a lot of stress!

7.   Do Only What's Important. Ultimately, the best way to help yourself avoid burnout is to listen to that little voice within you that tells you when enough is enough. If you think you may have too heavy a workload, write down all that you need to do and mark those items that are most important. What's left will have to wait, or will have to be done by someone else.

8.   Vent Your Emotions. If you start to feel the anxiety rising, take a deep breath or a short walk in order to clear your head. It's important that you express your emotions and not keep them bottled up inside. You can vent privately, to the bathroom mirror or in a journal, or you can release your frustrations with a friend. A notable source of burnout is unexpressed anger and emotion.

These burnout-stopping tips may help you enjoy your life again. Put these strategies into action now and before long, you'll be liberated from the overwhelming effects of burnout!

Chapter 5
Burnout Relief Strategies

Are you suffering from burnout? Whether it's caused by work issues, stress at home, relationship challenges, or a combination of all them, it can cause a frightening feeling of hopelessness!

Burnout often causes a feeling of numbness and not knowing how to get your life headed back in the right direction.

Take heart - hope is not lost! There *are* some strategies you can utilize to overcome burnout, once and for all.

Try these techniques to get relief from burnout:

1. **Don't blame yourself.** Life is hectic and stressful, especially with all the intense demands placed on our shoulders. If you're feeling burnt out, rather than blaming yourself, be proactive in getting back in the saddle so you can feel like yourself again.

- *Remember, you're in control of your destiny.* Focus on what you *can* do, not what you *think* you should do.

2. **Stop being so serious.** With the stress and responsibilities you carry on a daily basis, you may be in need of some *plain ol' silly time*. Release your inhibitions and have some fun!

- Whether it be dancing in your living room or swinging on the swings at a local park, take some time to find your inner child again. This will help you let go of your current stress level, even if it's just for a little while.

- *Making time to have fun will give you a chance to refocus and get your life and priorities back to where they need to be.*

3. **Stay healthy.** It's important to stay in peak physical condition when you're under constant stress. Eat many servings of fruits and vegetables, drink large amounts of water, and exercise.

• *Fit exercise into your busy schedule by making an appointment with yourself to exercise,* and then keep your appointment!

4. **Improve your time management skills.** You may be burnt out because you're trying to fit a week's worth of *stuff* into a single day. Unfortunately, that's impossible! Learning how to budget the time in your day more effectively will relieve a lot of this time pressure and stress.

• Good time management will lessen the feeling of being overwhelmed, as well as enable you to have the time you need to do what you want to do.

5. **Get enough sleep.** This allows your body to rest, rejuvenate, and start the upcoming day with more energy. You can also deal with stressful situations better when you're alert and focused.

• If you adhere to the 8 hours per night rule, you'll find yourself more focused, levelheaded, and patient.

No matter how you may try to sugar coat it, modern life isn't easy. It's no wonder that sometimes we feel like we can't juggle everything any more!

Although these feelings are normal from time to time, they can escalate out of control.

Before we reach that point, it's important to get our lives back in the right direction. These burnout strategies and tips will enable you to better handle every-day stresses so you can enjoy all the amazing gifts life has to offer!

Chapter 6
Prevent Burnout with Simple Strategies from Psychologists

Burnout can happen at any time to anyone, so it's important to prevent it. ***Psychologists have simple strategies for recognizing issues that can lead to burnout and giving you methods to deal positively with them.***

Burnout is a state that is best described as complete exhaustion. You may feel as if the world is ending, and you're completely overwhelmed by everything and everyone. Burnout can occur at work or at home.

Try these techniques to stop burnout in its tracks:

1. **Find a creative outlet.** Creativity is one of the best ways to prevent burnout.

- Do you have a creative outlet you can use to make your life easier? Do you love to draw, paint or play the piano?

- ***It's important to find a creative way to release energy and fight stress.***

2. **Find time for yourself.** Do you spend all of your time working and taking care of family or friends?

- It's crucial to find time for yourself in your busy schedule. ***Carve out some time each day to relax and do something you enjoy.*** Chores, work, family obligations, and everything else can wait.

- One of the main reasons burnout happens is because people keep pushing themselves and don't take enough breaks to regroup and heal.

- Psychologists recommend spending some time away from your to-do list. For example, you may want to eat lunch away from your desk in a more relaxing environment that truly gives you a break.

3. **Reach out to others.** Prevent burnout by talking about your concerns or worries with others. Do you have someone you can trust, so you can share the issues that weigh you down?

- *Communicating your concerns can help you discover new solutions to your challenges.* The support a friend or loved one provides can help you avoid burnout.

- It's tempting to avoid others during a burnout, but talking about the issues can help you solve them faster.

4. **Dig deep into your mind and soul.** Look inward. Why are you burning out? What is truly causing the stress in your life? It's important to look inside instead of just focusing on external issues.

- Are you being a perfectionist? Are you taking on too much work or home responsibilities? Evaluating your life can lead to crucial burnout solutions.

5. **Focus on the positive.** *Burnout can occur because your focus is lost and misdirected to negative emotions and thoughts.*

- Consider your daily thoughts and feelings. Are you focusing on the negative aspects of every situation? How can you change this, so your thoughts are on a more positive path?

- You may want to create lists of positive actions and thoughts throughout the day to stay on track. You can keep a notebook of inspirational ideas to help you avoid negativity.

- It's important to recognize negative emotions and what causes them before burnout occurs. You may have to set boundaries with people who are creating the negativity in your life. You may have to say no more often and reject more work or responsibilities to stay balanced.

• By focusing on the positive, you can reconsider your life goals.

You can prevent burnout by following the advice of psychologists and taking time to relax. Put these tips to use each day and you'll feel better sooner than you think!

Chapter 7
The Aftermath of Burnout: How to Rejuvenate Yourself

If you've recently suffered burnout, you'll likely be looking for ways to restore your peace, health, and happiness. It's important to treat yourself lovingly after such a trauma to your system so you don't develop chronic health conditions.

Burnout can cause all sorts of mental and emotional issues, including anxiety and depression. You should try to recognize the signs that lead to burnout, but this may not always be possible. If you concentrate on restoring yourself after burnout, you can avoid these issues and get your true self back.

Consider these burnout tips to help you regain your strength:

1. **Find a new direction.** The best, most permanent, way of dealing with burnout is to focus on making sustainable life changes. Ask yourself whether or not you're happy in your current situation. Perhaps it's time to make a major life shift, such as a new career or downsizing your home.

2. **Take a break.** It's best to get away from the situation that has caused you to burn out. This may mean going out for a walk and getting away for a few hours, or it may mean giving yourself a full blown vacation. You don't necessarily have to spend a lot of money for a vacation. Your goal is to relax and clear your mind. You can certainly do this at home or in your local community.

3. **Solve the problem.** If you're currently in the middle of a stressful situation, take action to solve the problem right away as best as you can. Consider the possible solutions to the problem and ask for help from others if necessary.

4. **Gain control.** Take control of the situation where possible. Realize that you can solve your problems and you're not doomed to remain in this state forever. Also, have the wisdom to accept that there are situations that are beyond your control. Do what you can to improve your situation, but avoid worrying about the things out of your control.

5.   Be open and honest. Sometimes it's best to set your pride aside and ask for help when you need it. Open up about the issues you're facing with a close friend or relative. If that's not an option for you, seek the help of a counselor.

Stress Management
If burnout tends to be a common occurrence for you, it would be in your best interest to start studying some stress management techniques.
There are certain things you can do to combat stress:
- Don't take on too much at work or at home.
- Remember that you can – and should – tell people "no."
- Make time for yourself.
- Ask for help from others.

Know Your Warning Signs
Once you've suffered burnout, you'll certainly want to know how you can avoid a similar situation in the future. Study the factors that led to burnout, and identify your mistakes so you can avoid making them again in the future.

These strategies will help you regain peace with yourself. If there are any outstanding issues that you need to resolve, seek solutions so you can achieve peace. You can do so through self-reflection, prayer, meditation, and communication. And once you do, you'll avoid burnout altogether!

Chapter 8
Understanding Burnout Associated with the Workplace

Burnout associated with the workplace is a common issue. This is normally a result of stress that is experienced in the workplace. When an employee suffers from work-related burnout, they often feel as if they are emotionally and mentally exhausted. In addition to this, it is also quite common to experience a true, physical exhaustion as well. When this common experience appears in an individual's life, a general sense of apathy may overwhelm them. They may feel disheartened and lack the motivation to perform even their basic responsibilities. Here, you will gain an understanding regarding burnout in the workplace.

When an individual experienced work-related burnout, it is a condition that has developed over time. It is not likely that an employee will become overwhelmed with burnout overnight. This is mostly a slow process that develops more and more as time progresses. This is a direct result of stress that is experienced in the workplace. Deadlines, dealing with uncooperative co-workers, unfavorable work conditions, and personal unhappiness in the work environment can all lead to burnout. This condition can affect all areas of an individual's life - job performance, relationships in the workplace, personal relationships, and even a person's health.

There are many signs and symptoms associated with work-related burnout. If you are in charge of employees, it is important that you gain an understanding of these signs. If you are an employee in the workplace, you should also learn the signs and symptoms associated with burnout. The more quickly that you are able to recognize that burnout is becoming evident, the quicker you can work to resolve the issues that you are facing. Listed below are some of the most common signs and symptoms associated with this common, and every real issue:

- One of the first signs of burnout is when an individual becomes frustrated. This frustration may be self-directed, directed to others, or towards the company in which they work.

- The second sign that an employee may be experiencing burnout is when their performance starts to falter. In many cases, this sign may be the most evident. A once reliable individual who completed work in a timely fashion that displayed a high level of quality may begin to take longer completing tasks, and the quality of their work may decline rapidly.

- Many individuals who experience workplace burnout may start expressing the fact that they feel as if they are "trapped" in their work situation. If an individual feels "trapped", this is a bad sign. It is important to be happy and content with the work that we do. If we feel anything else than this, it is important to seek assistance as workplace burnout is becoming evident.

- Those that experience this common work-related issue may start to detach themselves from friends, relatives, co-workers, social situations, and more. Social detachment is not a good sign. This is especially true when an individual is normally not socially withdrawn from others.

- Many who experience workplace burnout may seem extremely irritable. This may show in the means of rapid moods, and similar situations. If there is no apparent cause for this type of personality change, the issue may be related to workplace change.

- Many individuals may feel as if there is no hope for their current situation. They may walk in and out of each and every single day feeling a lack of motivation; many individuals may witness this behavior in the workplace and realize that it is uncharacteristic of the individual. This is a probable sign of work-related burnout.

- If you feel as if you have absolutely no power, you are not getting anywhere, and you find yourself constantly feeding negative thoughts and emotions, you may be experiencing workplace burnout.

- Many individuals who experience burnout often start experiencing many different kinds of failures. These failures may be directly related to their work performance, or they may be experienced in their personal life.

There are a number of causes that may lead an individual to experience burnout associated with the workplace. The following reasons may be associated with this type of work-related stress:

- Many individuals set their goals in the workplace too high. Setting high goals or having others in the workplace too high of goals is a common factor in workplace burnout.

- Many individuals may feel as if they are stuck in a particular job because they are unable to afford a change in careers, or they are unable to pass up the benefits that a job poses. For these individuals, workplace burnout may be experienced.

- Many individuals who have proved to be dependable and provide a high quality of work may be expected to consistently ask to perform additional work on top of their standard responsibilities. While many are flattered by the fact that they are given more work, this work can often become exhausting.

- There are many who do not feel personally challenged by their work. This type of work can become dull and a person may not feel as if they have anything to look forward to. This can result in workplace burnout as well.

Workplace burnout is a common issue that must be dealt with. If you are in charge of employees, it is important to know and understand the basics of workplace burnout. If you are an employee, it is important that you know and understands the basics as well. By understanding the conditions that cause this to occur, the symptoms associated with the condition, and how to overcome it, you can beat work-related burnout!

Chapter 9
Are You Suffering from Workplace Burnout?

Burnout is a state or condition where one experiences fatigue, exhaustion, or frustration as a result of an intense focus on our attention to a goal, a cause, a lifestyle or a relationship that fails to produce the expected reward. In other words, there is a burnout formula: expectations divided by a reality that does not meet your expectations, regardless of the effort you expend, equals burnout. There is no direct correlation or relationship between hard work and burnout. There is, however, a direct correlation or relationship between hard work that produces little or no reward, and burnout. In fact, many folks do actually work to exhaustion and they do achieve recognition, and reward. For these folks, burnout is not a part of the equation.

Am I Experiencing Burnout?

Burnout is a slow burn. Burnout is not an event; it's a process. Burnout is similar to erosion. One day you view a huge boulder under the waterfall. One day you return and it's half its original size. Then one day it's become a small stone; then a pebble. Burnout is an insidious and pernicious internal erosion.

Early symptoms of burnout include a deep sense of fatigue, tiredness, or exhaustion that seems to extend from the surface of your skin, through the tissues, ligaments, muscles, and deep into your bones and into the very cells of your body. Emotionally, you feel you are at or near the end of your emotional rope. Psychically, you live in a realm of negativity - experiencing a sense of dread, helplessness, hopelessness, negativity, cynicism or frustration. Relationships in and out of work suffer, They become exhausting; they are no longer fun and enjoyable. Work, itself, becomes an effort. Concentration is challenging. Staying focused is a formidable challenge. You feel and become detached, maybe even unattached from work and from the people in your life.

In the extreme, burnout manifests as an "uncaring" about life in general, about work life, family life....life. In the extreme, one cannot even muster the energy of anger, or resentment, or frustration; there is no energy, period. No feeling on any level (mental, emotional, physical, psychological, or spiritual). Just a numbness. Exhaustion. Life itself. becomes a huge effort.

Curiously, burnout affects folks who once felt alive, enthusiastic, excited, energetic, juicy, passionate and wonderfully curious about life and living. The upshot is their intention, passion and efforting to reach unattainable goals destroyed them in the process.

Organizations as the Cause of Burnout

All too often individuals believe they are the sole cause of their burnout. They feel they somehow are at fault for not being able to achieve work-life balance, or harmony in the way they live, or their inability to plan, organize, prioritize, schedule and execute or their efforting to be a 10 on a scale of 1-10, in everything they do, or because they are working for a manager whose expectations are exceedingly high and demanding. Sometimes, folks can be their own worst enemy and the cause of their own burnout. But, not always.

In fact, recent research is indicating that companies and businesses are often one of the worst causes of burnout. Burnout today is often built into the organizational structure. How so? Some of the organizational characteristics that lead to burnout are: impossible goals, countless layers of bureaucracy and just-plain-stupid policies and procedures, lack of clarity in roles and responsibilities, cloudy and confusing goals, endless and pointless meetings, and a pure "this is a business" mentality that focuses on people as functions while leaving the "human element" out of the equation.

So, at work, people begin to experiencing burnout when they feel they're in a "no-win" environment - that they'll never achieve no matter how long and how hard they keep working. Burnout happens when the writing on the wall spells "impossible" and "irrational", when there is no honest or logical rationale for the way business is conducted, for the way expectations are defined, for the way goals and results are determined, for the confusion about roles. When there is no connection between working hard and seeing the actual light at the end of the tunnel (i.e., results as well as "light" as in the form of "intelligence", "right action" and "meaning") folks become despairing, incredulous, and cynical.

One of the first behaviors that lead to burnout is confusion about what is expected. When responsibilities change from day to day, week to week, or month to month, burnout ensues. Folks end up competing against themselves. Workers become confused, foggy, frustrated and unhappy. They feel like they are swimming upstream. Soon, they begin to feel hopeless, helpless and exhausted. Burnout.

Another circumstance that creates burnout is having unclear role definitions, not having a clear idea of what expected of you. For example, an employee and their boss are not on the same page when it comes to the employee's role and responsibilities. Sometimes, this is a blind spot neither the employee or the boss is aware of. Each assumes what he or she knows to be true about the other. Soon the boss sees his/her expectations not being met and assumes the employee is incompetent, lazy or uninterested; in turn, the employee accuses their boss of being unfair, a bully or overbearing. Either way, there is a major disconnect that leads to frustration, resentment, and ill will. Burnout.

A third circumstance that leads to burnout is simple overload. Pushing added expectations, added tasks and added responsibilities on to an employee does not automatically mean the employee can handle the overload. More work does not produce better results. The manager often makes assumptions that

should not be made. When the employee takes on additional duties and becomes overloaded, the task load is not handled well. The result of overload is resentment and frustration. Burnout.

The Solution

If the issue is you and the way you work, the solution lies in your own hands. If it's your organization and its culture, you'll need to consider whether anything is likely to change. The final solution, simple, perhaps not easy, maybe to leave.

If you feel you're in the throes of burnout, your first action is to take time for your self, to engage in some deep self-reflection and look for root causes of the burnout issue. Then, consider the action steps to reduce or eliminate the degree of burnout you are experiencing.

Questions for self-reflection:

Do you have a pattern of taking on more work than you can handle? If so, why?

Does your boss continue to give you more work than you can reasonably handle? If so, have you spoken with your boss? With what result?

Do you ever feel helpless or hopeless at work? Frustrated, resentful? Why?

Is overload a cultural issue at your organization? Why? How did that come to be? Do managers and supervisors feel overloading is fair? How do they justify overloading employees?

Are you and your boss on the same page when it comes to their expectations of you and your expectations of you? If not, have you had a discussion with your boss about the inconsistencies? If not, why not?

If you're feeling burned out, are you aware that burnout can have serious, very serious, physical, mental, emotional and psychological repercussions........sooner rather than later? Is that OK? Are you choosing to let it be OK? Are you in denial about the burnout you are experiencing?

Do you feel you work hard with little to no reward? What action can you take to remedy this situation?

What one or two steps can you, or your organization, take this week and this month to reduce the intensity of the burnout you may be experiencing?

Reduce Stress and Prevent Burnout With the 3 R's - Review, Regroup, Renew! The 3 R's: Review, Regroup, Renew!

It is a privilege to be a wife, mother, daughter, sister, friend, and employee. These roles, however, should not replace the role of the individual. Many of us are pressured to make the most of our time each day. When we do have time to ourselves, we usually fill it with errands-housecleaning, laundry, grocery shopping, banking, etc. Our spouse, kids, parents, siblings, friends, and boss all take a piece of our day, but when was the last time you took time for you?

It's important for individuals to practice the three R's: review, regroup and renew! Eking out a few moments just for you is critical in order to maintain energy for the millions of things you do every day. Stress is cumulative. Without relief, it will build upon itself until you reach the final point of burnout. But you can stop this progression, and even reverse it, by simply taking time out for yourself. Individual "downtime" can help you put things in perspective, reduce stress, and prevent burnout. By taking care of yourself, you are better able to take care of others.

You don't have to schedule a week-long vacation in order to have some individual "down time". Let's face it, a family vacation is an antithesis of "down time".

Here are a few things you can do to rejuvenate and enjoy some "down time": Do absolutely NOTHING

One of my favorite songs is "Enjoy the Silence" by Depeche Mode. Kick off your shoes, sit in your favorite chair, relax your muscles and just breathe.

Get a massage or a facial

Get that kink out of your back and shoulders with a massage or relax with a soothing facial at the local spa.

Go on a "self" retreat

If you need to get away, but only have a day, fill the gas tank, grab a map and drive to a cozy little town or hop on the ferry for a day trip to a local island.

Make a date with yourself

Treat yourself to a gourmet meal for one at your favorite upscale restaurant. Chew slowly and savor every bite.

Take an art, dance, singing or music class

While signing your children up for classes, sign yourself up as well. Many programs offer separate classes for children and adults at the same time.

Cruise an art gallery or museum

Soak up the energy and appreciation of your fellow man's creative genius. Many museums and galleries offer free or discount days every month which will allow you to enjoy "down time" for little or nothing.

Chapter 10
Passive Income: Prevent Burnout and Enrich your Business

Service-oriented business owners sometimes struggle with not having enough hours in the day to tend to all the aspects of their business while generating sufficient income. Business owners can prevent burnout and enrich their business, by finding ways to create passive income.

Service providing business owners also face the risk of burning out if they take on a large case-load which demands large amounts of emotional, physical and mental energy. If you have a service-oriented business, much of your time is dedicated to quality interactions with clients and/or patients where you are fully engaged and fully present. You want to give your full attention to and use best practices with each client or patient and this can become draining if your caseload is too large.

Consider adding passive income. Passive income is a term used to refer to anything you are able to sell without being present to actually provide the service. I'll use my business as an example. Currently, I am splitting my time between small business coaching and counseling. My services require that I am face- to-face (or voice-to-voice via telephone) with my clients. When I am counseling or coaching someone, I want to be fully present and engaged, providing them with quality face-to-face time.

One way a coach, counselor, doctor, nutritionist, acupuncturist or any other service provider could make passive income while serving more people would be to develop some information products (DVDs, e- books, programs, etc.) that could be sold in an automated fashion online.

There are some individuals who may prefer to work through their life, health, relational or business challenges at their own pace and in the privacy of their home. They could do this by purchasing an information product or automated program. As a service provider, you would then be able to spread your energy around to all the aspects of your business without burning out. It would also allow you to enrich your business, serve more people, and create sufficient income to continue serving the world in your own unique way.

Give yourself permission to ponder what area of expertise you might be able to communicate through an information product or program in order to prevent burnout and enrich your business. I believe every individual has a unique area of knowledge or expertise that could be of help to a specific population or target audience. I would encourage you to take one step right now to research this possibility of creating passive income to prevent burnout and enrich your business.

Defending Against Personal Burnout and Frustration

Many leaders will associate the implementation of change in their organization with elevated levels of stress, frustration, and anxiety. These pressures, combined with a typical staff reduction that often requires leaders to accomplish more with less, can lead to personal burnout.

Change management, as incorporated in many organizational plans and strategies, often leads to personal burnout, as rather than take small, incremental steps that allow organizations to evolve. Many will stagnate and resist change until the company is severely threatened and must make huge, destabilizing adjustments to survive.

It is important for leaders to understand that large, overwhelming changes will typically shake up the entire organization as wholesale modifications occur in the way business is conducted. The process is time intensive and traumatic for everyone involved. People require time to recuperate after the event is over; wholesale changes often result in personal burnout.

Undoubtedly, quick and/or frequent change can lead to burnout. However, even in the face of ongoing change, leaders can use the strategies outlined in this section to defend against burnout and frustration.

Part of the Job

Effective leaders accept that change is a normal function associated with their jobs. In this way, change is no longer perceived as an event that threatens the organization, but simply a normal function of everyday business activity.

Leaders who embrace change plan small, incremental adjustments that help their organization slowly evolve and adapt. As a result, the company will eventually see an increase in productivity and efficiency. All it takes is a change in the leader's perception to reduce the stress and pressures that he or she once associated with organizational change.

Anticipate Rather Than Resist

When people oppose a change in their organization, they end up focusing their energy on resistance rather than acceptance. This focus saps the energy required to maintain productivity and effectiveness, which ultimately leads to burnout.

On the other hand, leaders who accept and anticipate change learn to harness its momentum to their benefit and use that energy to enact change throughout the organization, producing positive outcomes and results.

Pace

When organizations implement wholesale changes out of necessity, it can be overwhelming. Many of these changes include layoffs, which increase the intensity of the situation and overburden the leader. In turn, stress and anxiety levels go up, resulting in personal burnout.

However, when leaders plan for ongoing change, adjustments are made in small, incremental steps that allow the organization to transform itself on its own terms. Once done, wholesale organizational change is eliminated, as is the stress and intensity of change.

Incorporate

The incorporation of small, incremental changes into daily activities allows the organization to grow and evolve while simultaneously increasing productivity, effectiveness, and efficiency. The incremental nature of change allows leaders to build it seamlessly into the organizational culture.

When the organization accepts change as a daily occurrence, leaders don't really feel pressured nor do they experience high levels of personal stress and anxiety. This greatly reduces personal burnout.

Experiment

Leaders that learn to accept and incorporate change into their daily responsibilities also learn the value of experimenting with new ideas and concepts. They discover that small changes can be tested with minimal impact and that lessons can be learned from all successes and failures. These lessons are ultimately incorporated into adaptations made by the organization.

Experimentation also helps leaders reduce risks associated with change. And less risk equals less stress, frustration, and anxiety-all of which are associated with burnout.

Adrenal Burnout

Adrenal burnout has become a common disorder in today's stressed out, over-worked, emotionally exhausted society. As more and more people appear to suffer from perpetual fatigue, experiencing physical, mental, and chemical stress; affecting the body's chemistry on a cellular level and it is the cells in the adrenal glands that take the brunt of these stresses. All illnesses start with fatigue. The body is like a new car with power steering, power brakes, and power windows. When the power goes down, the entire car stops working right. Burnout is a serious medical problem, although symptoms may be vague and unrelated to a specific disease. The adrenal glands, which produce stress hormones, are affected by xenobiotic compounds (chemical compounds that are foreign to a living organism) more than any other organ.

Over the years, prolonged episodes of stress can cause the adrenals to become fatigued and are unable to regulate all the constituents of a healthy body. Sometimes the adrenals, in a weakened state, are referred to as insufficient, and as the progression of adrenal breakdown continues, it leads to adrenal burnout as termed by the late Dr. Paul Eck who researched adrenal function and tissue analysis for decades.

Adrenal Burnout is a very debilitating malady that can cause life-changing disruption. In severe cases, the adrenal activity is so acutely diminished that people have difficulty getting out of bed for more than a few hours per day. In each increment of reduction in adrenal function, every organ and system in the body is more profoundly affected. Changes can occur in the carbohydrate, protein and fat metabolism, fluid and electrolyte balance, heart and cardiovascular system, and even the sex drive.

Prolonged stress keeps the body in a constant and heightened fight or flight' state; if allowed to continue it would eventually compromise the adrenal function. The adrenals are the glands that sit near the top of each kidney. The inner part (the medulla) secretes hormones, including adrenaline and corticosteroid that control blood pressure, heart rate and sweating. They also act as chemical messengers; initiate immune responses; regulate blood sugar levels and produce much of the digestive juices used in breaking down foods. As they respond to stress the hormones raise blood sugar and blood pressure, and promote energy production. Adrenalin or epinephrine are used in emergencies when the adrenals become depleted, the body is unable to handle stress and this can lead to serious illness.

Symptoms of adrenal burnout can be weight gain, chronic infection especially respiratory problems such as influenza, bronchitis or pneumonia; impaired digestion, allergies, high blood pressure; high and low blood sugar levels, cravings for sweets; multiple chemical sensitivities, PMS; irritability and depression and even anxiety may occur.

The condition is also called adrenal hypofunction, exhaustion or insufficiency. Unlike fatigue, energy levels do not return after a good nights rest; it is a common misconception that the body is unable to regenerate energy during slumber; waking up tired after 8-10 hours of sleep is a primary symptom of burnout, like a dead battery, the body cannot recharge itself during sleep. Burnout is a more serious derangement of the body's energy system.

Adrenal burnout syndrome is rarely diagnosed by physicians and can be wrongly identified as Addison's disease which doctors consider incurable. However, recovery from adrenal burnout is definitely possible.

Burnout can develop slowly or may be caused by a single trauma. It was famously noted that John F. Kennedy experienced burnout during World War II when his patrol boat was rammed by a Japanese destroyer, killing most of the crew. He never recovered from the shock. For the rest of his life, he needed replacement adrenal hormones. If he had found the right practitioner, perhaps they would not have been needed.

A disproportionate amount of stress can be an important cause of burnout which can be derived from many sources. Chemical toxicity and nutritional depletion are among the physical causes; Mental, emotional or spiritual stress can be a major factor and overwork, financial and family problems; noise in

the cities and electromagnetic pollution; mobile phones, microwave towers, and household or workplace appliances that emanate strong electrical fields.

Nutritional Deficiencies are also a common cause. When the body is under stress, there is a greater need for nutrients. Carbohydrates, when excessive in the diet, stress the adrenals. Diets low in protein may also create deficiencies. Inadequate or poor quality water affects the oxygenation of the tissues.

Most diets are deficient in nutrients that are required by the adrenals. These include B-complex vitamins, vitamins A, C and E, manganese, zinc, chromium, selenium and other and other trace elements. The majority of cheap supermarket food in today's consumer society is grown in depleted soils. Further processing and refining reduce nutrients even more. Bad habits like eating in the car or while on the run can further diminish the value derived from food. Also, allergic reactions to foods such as wheat and dairy products can damage the intestines and reduce the absorption of nutrients.

Toxic metals and chemicals can also contribute to adrenal burnout; as exposure to a multitude of chemicals in the air, water and food are becoming increasingly prevalent in today's society. Dental materials; skin contact with chemicals; over-the-counter and prescribed medications are also conducive to the body's toxic load.

Toxins can be generated within the body due to impaired digestion. When food is not properly digested, it either ferments or rots in the intestines, producing many harmful substances that are absorbed back into the body.

Chronic infections can also purvey to the toxic load. For many, the elimination organs refrain from functioning at optimal levels; resulting in a build-up of toxic substances within the body; leading to adrenal burnout and many other health conditions.

Many stimulants such as caffeine, sugar, and alcohol can damage the adrenals as they incite the glands into action. Less obvious stimulants can include anger, rage, arguing, hatred, loud music, the news and movies full of suspense; vigorous exercise, sexual preoccupations and the use of stimulants. Artificial stimulants can appear alluring in the midst of fatigue, providing a temporary energy surge or buzz. It is an appeal of the drug culture, both legal and recreational.

Unhealthy responses to stress such as worrying, becoming angry or afraid can induce a burnout. Particularly high strung, nervous individuals and those with very active minds are especially prone to adrenal burnout. Unfortunately, many with adrenal burnout function on anger and resentment. These act as adrenal stimulants, providing a negative energy with which to function.

Secondary to adrenal exhaustion are glandular imbalances, hyperthyroidism and more often hypothyroidism. The adrenal glands produce estrogens and progesterone, the main source of hormones

post-menopause. Premenstrual syndrome and hot flushes are also indicative of weakened adrenal glands.

The side effects of adrenal burnout can be depression and apathy to friends, family, and work. Anxiety and Irritability can also occur, as the inability to handle even minor stresses confounds. Compulsiveness and OCD are also associated; precipitating addictions of excessive exercise, sex, loud music or other forms of excitement. The unconscious goal is always the same, to stimulate the adrenals into activity.

When the adrenals are weak, copper builds up in the body. Elevated copper enhances emotions. Panic attacks, bipolar disorder, mood swings and schizophrenia are related to copper imbalance. As energy levels decline, other toxic metals build up as well. Mercury, cadmium, lead, arsenic, beryllium, and others contribute to hundreds of physical and emotional symptoms. Elevated copper and low zinc levels can impair the immune system and chronic infections can occur. The stage is also set for the development of degenerative conditions such as Cancer, heart disease, Parkinson's and Alzheimer's diseases are end-stage results of toxic accumulation and energy depletion

The condition can be classed as psychological as stress engenders the burnout which in turn affects the emotions and behavior. But, burnout is biochemical as recovery involves improving emotions and dealing with psychological issues. However, it also involves rebuilding body chemistry because it is a physical condition as well.

Adrenal burnout is more prevalent among women than men; mainly due to lifestyle changes and sluggish oxidization rates. However, it is just as common in men. Many children are also born with weak adrenals due to their parents' nutritional deficiencies. Minimal brain dysfunction, chronic ear or other infections, crib death, failure to thrive, ADHD and anti-social behavior may all be symptoms of burnout in children.

Burnout can occur in all groups in society, regardless of occupation, income or educational level. It is recognized that many homeless people are victims of burnout. Accounting for why they may give up hope or be incapable of holding a job or supporting a home. Burnout affects every area of life; family, work, and relationships; apathy everyone and everything. Friends, family, and employers are often unaware of the condition, which can exacerbate the situation.

Burnout can occur due to a single shock; traumas that occur together or a combination of factors. Whether it is derived from an illness, accident, divorce, overwork or other stress depends very much on one's ability to handle stress, rather than the absolute amount of stress. When the burnout manifests, vital minerals can become depleted and toxic substances replace and become part of the structure of enzymes, body organs, and glands. Even after a change of diet, lifestyle, attitudes or behavior, the toxins can remain.

Often, burnout does not even develop until several years after a trauma, illness or injury as depleted and damaged cells proliferate. Even though many change their diets and get over their traumas, most people never recover from burnout or make only a partial recovery.

The accumulation of toxins that occurs as the body and the inability to eliminate them can contribute to burnout. Elimination is very important, however, energy is required to release toxins. If the energy system is weak, just fasting or cleansing will not be enough. One must rebuild the entire energy system by balancing body chemistry and providing nutrients as well. A one-month or even six-month cleanse is nowhere near adequate. It can take a year just to replenish one mineral. For those in burnout, extreme detoxification programs such as fasting, raw foods or even chelating agents can be dangerous. This is because the body lacks the vitality to properly eliminate toxins, the eliminative organs are compromised and toxins may be redistributed in vital organs. A gentle, complete program of rebuilding and nourishing the body must accompany any efforts to eliminate toxins. In fact, as vitality improves, toxin elimination will proceed of its own accord.

Diet is an extremely important factor in the road to recovery. Protein should be eaten with every meal, eggs, natural meats, and poultry are among the best sources; toasted almond butter, goat's cheese, and nuts are other alternatives. It is advised to avoid vegetarian diets. At meal times try and east at least three different vegetables; it is advised to rotate proteins and vegetables, so as not to consume the same thing every day.

Complex carbohydrates are allowed but wheat and spelt should be avoided as sensitivities to gluten (found in rye, barley, and oats) can occur. Excellent starches are root vegetables (turnips, parsnips, rutabaga, carrots, onion and celery root), blue corn, brown rice, quinoa and others.

It is recommended to reduce all sweets and fruit. Avoid sugar and cows milk dairy products (except butter); vegetable oils except for olive oil; isolated soy protein as it is of poor quality and contains many anti-nutrients; junk food; juices as they can be too sugary and can concentrate food toxins, upset blood sugar levels and weaken the adrenals. Use sea salt rather than table salt; eat regular meals of an excellent quality and switch to organic food whenever possible.

Green foods like kelp, barley grass powder, and various colored vegetables are highly recommended. Cooking with coconut oil is excellent as it aids weight loss, Candida Albicans infection, and energy. It is also advised to drink high-quality water such as distilled or spring and to avoid tap water.

Chapter 11
Why You Must Stress Less

We all know that stress is bad for us and this is something we get told very often. However, it's all too easy to write this off as being a minor nuisance or frustration rather than anything to really worry about. We all get stressed from time to time, right?

In reality though, this is the wrong way to think about stress. While it is fairly common place, that is not to say that it isn't serious. In fact, stress is *incredibly* serious and can cause severe problems both in the short term and long term.

Stress can shorten your lifespan. Ruin your enjoyment. Cause serious illness. Shrink your brain. Hurt your performance. Ruin your relationships. Cause impotence.

Do those sound like small matters?

To understand this better, it can help to look more closely at what precisely stress is. *How* it causes the problems it does and how and why you need to do everything you can to prevent and reduce it.

So What Exactly is Stress?

Stress is what we feel when we're overworked, when we're dreading something that's about to happen or when we're generally unable to relax and stay calm due to outside or inside factors influencing our thoughts.

But it actually goes beyond this. Stress is a basic physiological reaction that is designed to help us focus and survive. In itself it is not a bad thing and is actually rather adaptive. The problem is that it has been taken out of context, which means the positive effects become outweighed by the negative.

Essentially, stress is what causes the 'fight or flight response'. This is a physiological response to perceived danger, designed to improve our chances of survival. If you were to see a lion for example, this would trigger a cascade of effects collectively resulting in the stress response.

This begins when we observe danger or experience fear. Increased activity in our brain, causes the release of adrenaline, as well as dopamine, norepinephrine and cortisol – our stress hormones. These then trigger a number of physiological changes: increasing our heartrate, making us breathe more quickly and making us more acutely focussed on the potential threat.

<u>A list of the symptoms should include:</u>

• Increased heartrate

• Rapid, shallow breathing

• Muscle contraction

• Tunnel vision

• Heightened sensitivity

• Increased blood viscosity

• Suppression of the pain response

• Suppression of the immune system

• Suppression of the digestive system

• Dilation of the pupils

• Dilation of the blood vessels

In the short term, this is good for us. In the short term, these things help us to evade danger and win combative situations. Increased muscle tension makes us stronger. Increased blood viscosity makes our blood more likely to clot in case of an injury. Dilated pupils let more light in to improve our vision. Suppression of secondary functions means that more blood can be sent to the muscles and the brain. Reduced pain means we can carry on fighting or running despite injury.

In short, anything that can help you to survive is prioritized, while secondary functions are suppressed. The idea is that once we get to safety, we can then turn off this fight or flight response and instead enter the 'rest and digest' state in order to recover. Once the predator is gone, we can recover.

But the problem is that in our modern environments, predators aren't the main problem. It's rare these days for us to be chased, to get into a fight or to need to escape a forest fire.

What's *not* so rare, is for our boss to shout at us and to tell us that we're late for our deadline. It's not rare for us to be in debt. It's not rare for us to have marital problems.

And unfortunately, the brain interprets all these signals in just the same way: as threats. And this causes the same fight or flight response. But because these types of threats aren't so easily resolved, this means we'll often end up on heightened alert for a longer period of time.

This is also why stress causes impotence in men. If you are highly stressed, blood is sent *everywhere* except the genitals!

And this takes a tremendous toll on our bodies.

As you might imagine: it is not good for you when your immune system and digestive system are suppressed for days. It's also not good for your brain to be flooded with norepinephrine and cortisol. It's not good for your heartrate to stay elevated, or your blood pressure to stay high.

This is the problem with *chronic* stress as opposed to acute stress. And it's the problem with heightened levels of stress, as opposed to the gentle, motivating force of 'eustress'. We'll look at all of this more in the long term, but suffice to say that the longer stress like this continues, the more you start to feel drained, malnourished, fatigued, ill and possibly eventually depressed.

How Stress Damages the Brain

When we are stressed, it effectively makes us less intelligent. This is due to the reduction in pre-frontal activity, which in turn is designed to make us more focussed and alert. Essentially, the pre-frontal cortex is the part of the brain responsible for forward planning, creative thinking and other 'high-order' brain activity.

When you are being chased by a lion though, it is really not the time to be thinking about the meaning of life!

So shutting down this part of the brain and placing your focus on feedback from your senses makes much more sense.

Of course that's not particularly useful in the workplace though: and this is why the stress response is so seriously *un*helpful when we have to give a presentation, answer a question on the spot or go on a date. This is when we lose all articulation and start stammering and saying useless things.

Slightly longer-term is adrenal fatigue. This is what happens when your brain has exhausted its supply of adrenaline and other stress hormones. That might sound like a good thing but you actually need a little norepinephrine, dopamine and cortisol to stay motivated – and even to wake up in the morning! Adrenal fatigue leaves you listless, demotivated and potentially depressed. It can also cause what is known as 'learned helplessness' – a condition where you essentially completely give up because your brain has been conditioned to learn that any attempts to change its situation will be met with failure. Not good!

Worse, when you are highly stressed, it can lead to *long term* problems for your brain health. As we briefly mentioned: it can *literally* shrink your brain! Studies show that in the long term, it leads to structural changes that shrink the hippocampus and shrink grey matter – the all-important neural connections throughout the brain. Even a single, severe traumatic event can result in significant reductions in the medial PFC, anterior cingulate and subgenual regions of the brain. The effects of 'cumulative adversity' meanwhile, cause smaller volumes in the medial prefrontal cortex (the PFC), insular cortex and anterior cingulate regions.

These regions of the brain correspond with emotional control, decision- making, reasoning and self control.

In other words, the eventual result of stress is to leave you more reactionary, more depressive, more impulsive and less disciplined.

From here, *every* aspect of your life will start to see negative effects. But there are things you can do about it...

Chapter 12
How To Manage Normal Stress

Just understanding these factors, you can hopefully see that stress isn't a 'bad thing' necessarily: rather it is a useful and required part of a normal, healthy, functioning body. In fact, as we've discussed, a little stress is necessary in order to help you feel more alert, more focussed and more productive. If we never had even a small amount of stress hormones in our system, then we would spend all our time highly rested and too laid back to get any actual work done!

The key is to make sure that those stress levels stay at this optimal level, as well as to try and get your natural cycles to line up with the times when you need to be most productive during the day.

And we can start by hijacking some of the physiological aspects we've already discussed...

Managing Blood Sugar

One very simple way to keep your stress at bay, is to avoid letting your blood sugar drop too low. We've already seen that low blood sugar triggers the release of cortisol and other stress hormones and so it follows that by avoiding low blood sugar, we can avoid this fate.

The best way to manage your blood sugar levels, is to avoid consuming simple carbohydrates. Carbohydrates are the best source of blood sugar for the human body but the problem is that in their 'simple' form, they release energy into the blood much too quickly. This results in a sudden spike in sugar, which then gets taken up and leaves you drained again. What's more, is that this causes the release of melatonin – the sleep hormone – as we've seen earlier. Not ideal for working.

If you have a breakfast that is made up of pancakes and syrup then, it will wake you up and make you feel good in the morning but an hour later you'll start to run low on energy and that will cue the release of cortisol.

So instead, try consuming a source of calories that will release the sugar more gradually into your bloodstream. A great choice is some form of complex carbohydrate, such as oats. This takes longer to reach the blood stream, providing a steady stream of blood sugar and preventing you from going into alert 'starvation' mode.

Conversely, fat will also have the same effect. When you consume a saturated fat, this will once again sit in the stomach while it gets broken down, providing you with a steady release of energy that will help you go about your business throughout the day.

Stay Comfortable

Comfort is fantastic for reducing stress and this has been shown in studies to help boost creativity. It only takes your keys to be digging into your pocket for example, for your body to consider you as uncomfortable and potentially being damaged. Thus, you will find that if you can sit in a more supportive and comfortable chair and also ensure the temperature is right and you are surrounded by things that put you at ease (plants have been shown to do this well for most people), then you will start to feel a lot calmer – even when you're at work and other stresses are being thrown at you.

Spend Time Away From Screens

Computers, smartphones and television are all great. They're entertaining and they're great for productivity. Unfortunately though, they're also very bad for us when it comes to stress hormones. We've already discussed how light from screens can trigger the release of cortisol and we've seen that the constant messages and alerts essentially trigger a series of small stress responses while we're surfing the web.

This is manageable but it becomes problematic when you spend too much time on the computer. Simply going for occasional walks and taking breaks from the screen throughout the day then will be a great way to help your body recover.

Another tip is to take time off just before bed. If you aim to have a restorative and restful night's sleep, then you need to give yourself time to 'wind down' just before you hit the sack. Taking time away from computers is one of the best ways to do this, so why not have a bath before bed with some candles instead? Or read by a more natural type of light? Give yourself half an hour of 'screen off' time and you'll find you get to sleep much quicker and feel more restored in the morning.

No can do? If you absolutely can't separate yourself from your gadgets at the end of the day, then try using software that will reduce the amount of 'blue light' coming from the screen. Redshift technology will help you block the most damaging wavelengths from your devices and thereby create a more restful light. An alternative is to wear 'blue blocking shades' which can block all blue light in your environment before bed!

Get Rid of Your Alarm

You know what really isn't helping your stress levels?

Your morning alarm!

The reason alarms tend to choose from a generic range of sounds, is that bleeps and ringing sounds are unnatural. These sounds don't occur in nature and thus we are attuned to them and they make us naturally sit up and take notice. In other words: they trigger a stress response.

And now bear in mind that when this happens, you are often in the very deepest stage of sleep. What a way to start your day! Rudely woken from the depths of sleep by a blaring noise, only to find yourself in a pitch dark room.

There are two much healthier alternatives to consider...

Fitness Tracker

One option is to use a fitness tracker/smart watch that has a smart alarm function. These work by monitoring your heartrate and your movement during the night, in order to estimate how awake or asleep you are at any given stage. Using this information, they can then wake you up at the point when you're in light REM sleep, rather than deep SWS sleep. The result is that you're woken at a point when you're already coming around anyway – and this is combined with a gentle nudge from a vibration, rather than a loud ringing.

Daylight Lamp

Better yet, is to use a daylight lamp. These are lamps that are designed to create a wavelength similar to that of the sun – with plenty of blue light! In that way, these are the opposite of redshift technology or blue blocking shades.

These lights will then be built into alarm, that are able to gradually get brighter as it nears the point that you set to wake up at. This helps to gradually stir you into wakefulness, by mimicking the effects of a sunrise. You start to feel more and more awake and your brain produces hormones associated with waking up – such as cortisol and nitric oxide.

While this is a stress response, it's a much milder and more natural stress response to the one that is caused by the sudden blaring of an alarm. The result is that you feel calmer and happier during the day and that you'll be better able to sustain levels of activity later thanks to a more accurate body clock.

Rethink Your Commute

Commuting to work is one of the worst things you can do for your stress levels throughout the day.

Did you know for example, that a typical commute will trigger huge amounts of what is considered to be the only 'universal fear'?

So what is this universal fear? It's things moving quickly toward you. Across all cultures and all demographics, moving something quickly towards a person's face will cause them to recoil and to see an increase in their heartrate and their stress response. Now think about a typical commute – filled with people moving rapidly towards you, lots of noise, lots of pollution and generally huge amounts of chaos. Before your day has even begun, you'll be experiencing huge amounts of stress.

This might be outside of your control. But if it *is* within your control, then make sure you do anything you can to avoid this kind of commute. Even just going in an hour earlier to avoid the rush-hour may be a good choice.

Rethink Your Morning Coffee

You know what else *really* isn't helping your stress in the morning?

That cup of coffee!

When you drink coffee, you are essentially experiencing the stress response in a cup. That's because coffee works by triggering something akin to a stress response.

It starts by mimicking a molecule we all have in our brains called 'adenosine'. Adenosine is a by-product of the energy systems in the body and it builds up over time as we are active. The more you use your brain power, the more of this substance accumulates.

The problem, is that adenosine is also an inhibitory neurotransmitter. The more adenosine builds up, the tireder we get and the less active the brain becomes. This is one of the reasons that we find ourselves feeling tireder and less cognitive able as the day drags on.

Drink caffeine though and the brain's 'adenosine receptors' get confused. They absorb caffeine instead of adenosine and this means the adenosine has nowhere to go and can't work. This in turn, gives you an instant boost in energy levels by making you feel more awake and focussed.

This also leads to a general increase in brain activity though and this is where the stress response comes in. The brain notices this sudden wakefulness and what do you know, it assumes that something very important must be going on. Thus, we see a release of more neurotransmitters associated with stress! Our good friends cortisol, norepinephrine, adrenaline and dopamine. This increases the heartrate, dilates the pupils, suppresses the immune system... all the things that any other stress response does.

Caffeine in itself is not bad. In small doses it can help boost memory and wakefulness and it's actually protective against all kinds of neurodegenerative diseases in the long term. But what it also is, is a quick way to make any stressful situation worse. If you've got a busy day, you just commuted during rush hour and you sit down at work to drink a big cup of coffee, you're only going to make yourself *more* stressed and wired.

And guess what? Once again, this is going to result in a crash shortly afterward when your energy levels have been depleted.

Don't drink caffeine as part of a routine. Drink it when you need that extra push – don't rely on it and don't combine it with other stress.

Chapter 13
Meditation

While all these changes can help, there is one thing that is more powerful than any other tool when it comes to combating stress: meditation.

Meditation is something a lot of people don't fully understand. There is the assumption among some that meditation is somehow 'mystical' or that it is necessarily linked with religion. Neither of these things is true.

There are many different types of meditation from transcendental, to mindfulness, to religious meditation but all of them really just have one thing in common: they involve the purposeful direction of attention inward.

Whether it is reflecting on your own thoughts, praying or just sitting silently and trying to clear your mind, meditation involves making the conscious decision to take control of what you're thinking and to try and stop your thoughts from jumping around everywhere. And when you do this, you will find it has a truly profound effect on your ability to stay calm in stressful situations, to control the nature of your thoughts and to combat many of the negative effects of stress.

In fact, studies show us that meditation can improve the areas of your brain that stress destroys – actually increasing the amount of grey matter in the brain and the amount of whole-brain connectivity. Furthermore, it can help to improve areas of the brain specifically related to motivation, attention and willpower. One study shows that it only takes 8 weeks to see amazing positive changes to the brain and restoration of grey matter in particular.

People who use meditation will usually report that they feel generally calmer, happier and more at peace throughout the day.

This results in a better mood, heightened attention and general improvements in cognitive function and productivity.

All these things mean that meditation is actually the perfect antidote to stress and can undo a lot of the damage that meditation causes. Apart from anything else, meditation will help you to take a small break from the constant stress of daily life and from the racing thoughts that come with this. More to the point though, it will teach you to take control of racing thoughts at will and simply to put them to one side.

Meanwhile, allowing your brain some time to enjoy this highly relaxed state will encourage the reparation of neurons and the cementing of things you've learned through the day.

Finally, it makes sense that areas controlling self-control would develop during the process of meditation. Meditation uses certain brain areas and we now know that the more you use an area of the brain, the more it grows. This works just like using a muscle and is a process known as 'brain plasticity'.

And by practicing reflecting on your own mental state and being more aware of your own emotions, it only follows that you would better be able to control it and to avoid letting stress or impulse get the better of you in future.

How to Get Started With Meditation

So this is what meditation does for you and why it is the ideal antidote to stress.

The next question is how can you get started with meditation? Do you need to attend a class? Do you need to be a Buddhist monk?

Fortunately, meditation is actually pretty simple and this is what ends up making it hard even in some cases. A lot of people who first try meditation feel that it is *too* simple and thus assume they must be doing something wrong!

The easiest way to get started if you're a complete beginner, is to try guided meditation. Guided meditation means using a pre-recorded script that will talk you through everything you need to be doing at any given stage. Essentially, this works to help direct your attention and show you what you need to be reflecting on or paying attention to at any given time.

A good one to try is 'Headspace'. This is available as a website and as an app and in either case, you'll find a selection of guided meditations to walk you through. The only downside is that headspace is not free and that after the first 10 sessions, you'll have to start paying.

Fortunately, those first ten sessions are more than enough to give you a taste of meditation and to teach you the basics. From here, you'll then be able to take what you learned and re-apply it in order to continue on your own.

If you'd rather not start a paid system though, then you can always use one of the *many* free YouTube videos that will do the same thing!

In general, most guided meditation will take you through the following steps.

To start with, you will sit somewhere comfortable and close your eyes. Set a timer for 10 minutes, or however long you have until you need to be doing other things. While you should be comfortable, you shouldn't be too reclined or generally put yourself in danger of falling asleep!

The next thing to do, is to bring your attention to the sounds and the world around you. This means just listening to the sounds and noticing what you can hear. This is an interesting exercise in and of itself: if you actually stop to listen you'll be able to pick up on a *lot* more information than you were probably previously aware of.

Don't strain to listen but instead just let the sounds come to you – whether those be barks from dogs next door, the sound of birds or perhaps chatter from someone in another building that you can hear through the walls.

After you have done this for a little while, the next step is to bring your attention in to yourself and to notice how your body feels. This means noticing the way that your weight is distributed on your buttocks. Is it evenly distributed? Are you leaning slightly to one side? Likewise, try to notice the air against your skin, the temperature, any aches and pains etc.

You can then try the 'body scan'. This is something that some people use as the main basis for their meditation and it involves focussing on each part of your own body, starting right from the head and then moving down the body slowly from the face, to the chest, to the legs, to the feet. Each time you get to a point on your body, make a conscious effort to release any tension you might be holding there and to relax.

You can even turn your attention inward further by seeing if you can feel the beating of your own heart, or the movement of your diaphragm.

Either way, we're now going to focus on breathing. This is something that a lot of people will again use as the entire basis of their meditation. Simply count the breaths in and the breaths out and each time you get to ten, start again. The aim now is to have all of your focus and all of your attention on the breathing and not to be distracted by anything outside.

Now, from time to time, you will notice that your thoughts start to drift and that you end up thinking about other things. This is a fantastic example of just how hard we find it to focus on any one thing for a given period of time. It's a fantastic example of just why you *need* this meditation!

Don't fret when it happens though. This is the worst thing you can do! Instead, simply 'notice' that your mind has wandered and then bring your attention *back* to your breathing again. Each time it drifts off, just re-center and don't worry about it.

Focussing on the breathing is simply giving us a way to center our thoughts and to remove the distractions that normally interrupt. This could just as easily work by focussing on anything else: for example, some people will focus on a single word called a 'mantra'. A mantra is what is often used in transcendental meditation for instance and might mean just repeating the word 'Om' in order to busy your internal monologue.

Finally, the last stage of our guided meditation is going to be to just let the thoughts wander freely and to let them go wherever they want to.

This last stage is essentially mindfulness meditation. The idea is that you're going to detach yourself from those thoughts and simply 'watch them' rather than feeling emotionally affected by them.

This last part is the part where you get to really relax and stop 'fighting' your brain and it's a great way to end. Then bring your focus back to your breathing, then back to your body, back to the world around you and eventually open your eyes.

Congratulations, that was your first meditation session!

Tips

Learning to meditate and making it a part of your life are two very different things and a lot of people reading this are now going to struggle to adopt this new behavior in a meaningful way.

The first issue is that a lot of people get frustrated when they feel that their meditation isn't 'working' and they thus give up. This is entirely the wrong way to look at meditation – this is not a means to an end but rather a relaxing place you can come and visit whenever you need it, or a great interlude before you start your day.

This extends to how you start out. A lot of people want things to go perfectly right away and they'll wonder why they haven't achieved enlightenment as soon as they close their eyes! Then their hair gets in their face, they become stressed that they aren't doing it right and they get up. Then they need to itch. Then they're not comfortable.

Don't worry about it. It's fine to move. It's fine to open your eyes for a moment. All that's important is that you then bring your attention *back*. In time, you'll find you are less distracted. But to begin with, you won't be ready for that yet and you mustn't get frustrated when you find that distractions do arise.

The next tip is to think carefully about how you're going to sustain your meditation training and make it a feasible part of your routine. A lot of resources will tell you how easy it should be to take 10 minutes out of your day. They'll claim that 'everyone' has five minutes.

In reality though, it's *not* easy. If it were, then everyone would already be doing it! Most of us are so busy that we legitimately struggle to find five minutes of free time and so we need to be realistic about what we can and can't achieve.

Look at it this way: it's much better to practice for two minutes twice a week and actually *stick with it*, than it is to try and practice for an hour a day and to give up after day two.

The best thing to do is to find an opportunity when you waste time in the morning or the evening. This might be while your partner goes through the shower in the morning, or it might be when you get home from work. Whatever it is, most of us have a few short periods of time in our usual routine and the great thing about meditation is that you can do it anywhere and with no props. Even if it's on the train to work, or if it is when you get into work 10 minutes early. If you can find a 'slot' that already exists, you'll find it's much easier to fit meditation in and to stick with.

Correct Breathing for Stress Reduction

When meditating it is important to try to remember to breathe properly. And better yet is to try and make this into a habit so that your breathing is better during your waking day as well.

The thing is: a lot of people don't know *how* to breathe well and are unintentionally breathing incorrectly most of the time. Theory has it that the reason for this is closely linked to the way we sit at work.

This is a big deal if you're trying to reduce stress, seeing as your stress levels are closely related to the way you breathe. We've already seen that there is a strong connection between physiology, feelings, emotions and psychology. When we are stressed, we breathe more quickly and not as deeply. But likewise, when we breathe more quickly and not as deeply, we *become* more stressed.

Right now, take both hands and place one on your stomach and one on your chest. Now breathe normally. Which hand is moving first? Is it the hand on your chest or the hand on your stomach?

For most people, the answer is the chest. But to be optimally healthy, it should be the stomach. When we're infants this is how we breathe and it's also how animals breathe. Years of sitting in an office desk though, or on a sofa, mean that we've spent too long with our stomachs compressed and learned to breathe differently.

Stomach breathing means that you are relaxing your abdominal muscles, thereby opening up your abdominal cavity and allowing your diaphragm to drop down into that space. This then creates more room for the lungs and they will automatically inflate as they enlarge. You *then* bring your chest in and open that up to take in even more oxygen and as a result, you breathe a lot more deeply. This oxygenates your body and it calms your heartrate and helps you to feel less stressed.

In fact, one of the very best ways to help yourself feel instantly less stressed, is to start taking deep, controlled breaths. This puts you in a rest and digest state and stops the fight or flight response in its tracks. So if you're about to go to an interview or give a presentation, practicing some controlled breathing for a while is the perfect antidote to the stress you're probably experiencing.

Hopefully at this point, you have all the tools and knowledge you need to begin reducing and combating the stress in your own life.

This isn't going to be an easy ride. Stress for many of us has become a normal part of life and habits are hard to change.

But by using meditation, you'll find that you can reduce your base level of stress and rebuild some of the damage to your brain caused by anxiety. What's more, is that this will teach you to be more aware of your thoughts and better able to control them and thereby steer your emotions.

It's time to wrestle back control of your mind. *You* tell your body when it needs to wake up and when it needs to focus. You decide what's worth worrying about. And when you're home and work is over, you use this power to allow yourself to rest, recover and forget all about the stresses of the day.

Once you can do all this, you'll find your mood improves, your productivity skyrockets and your health is greatly enhanced in both the long *and* short term.

Stress less, live more.

Chapter 14
3 Top Ways To Reduce Everyday Stress

Learning how to deal with stress is something that everybody needs to know. Even our health can suffer the effects of stress which can also make it difficult to think clearly enough to solve even the simplest task. The good news is that there are simple easy techniques for reducing your stress which we will cover here in this article.

As more studies show the link between stress and many health problems, stress management becomes an important consideration for many people. These 3 top stress management ways can help you to reduce the levels of stress in your life, so make good use of them.

Massage

Go get a massage, this is the first method for reducing and managing stress levels. Massage has often been thought of as a great way to relieve sore muscles, but it can also reduce overall body tension, anxiety and stress too. There are a lot of studies that prove massage is a great way to reduce stress when done regularly. There are many different types of massage, so you should try several kinds and find the one that you prefer. Nowadays it's not usually hard to find qualified massage therapists. Massage can release endorphins in the brain which produce pleasure which is helpful in not only stress reduction but also helpful for emotional issues such as anxiety and depression to name a few.

Relaxation Techniques

We have all already probably heard of various methods of relaxation. Some of the most popular methods are basic mediation and the various forms of yoga. You can attend online or actual classes to learn the different parts of these methods so you can learn to relax. There are also other options to these major relaxation techniques. A simpler and more straightforward option would be to learn deep breathing techniques. You can use these even when you are seated in your work station. Progressive muscle relaxation and mental imagery are also possible basic techniques you can use against stress.

Exercising on Schedule

It's just like what your physical education teacher always said. Maintaining a regular exercise schedule can do wonders for your body. The major benefit of exercise is that it can encourage the proper circulation of your blood. This in turn ensures that oxygen and nutrients reach the various cells in your body. You need these if you ever hope to fight the bad effects of stress on your health.

You've now heard only a few of the most effective stress management tips available there are still other ways to approach the management of your overall stress including enough sleep and eating health. What causes your stress can be as important as treating it so you need to know what that is. Stress management can take many forms, and the methods you use will depend on your circumstances and what you prefer.

Chapter 15
How To Manage Anxiety and Panic Attacks

Everyone is susceptible to anxiety attacks, although they attack different people in varying degrees of intensity. Anxiety can greatly hinder one from doing a lot of things. Fear has a way of crippling a person's potential and robbing them of the chance to be at their very best. Luckily however, there are some simple things you can do to combat anxiety when it attacks without warning. Although there is no guarantee that the anxiety will completely go away, following the tips below will ensure that the anxiety levels do subside. Here is what to do when you feel the pangs of anxiety settling in:

Distract yourself for a while

It is impossible to calm yourself if you stay in the stressful situation for long. The very first thing to do is to distract your brain from the situation for a few minutes. This does not mean that you ignore it completely. You will have to confront your fears sooner or later, but you should give yourself a break from the panic- ridden situation for a while. Prepare your favorite meal. Listen to your favorite song. Or you could even take a brief walk. Just do anything that will take your mind off the situation for some time.

Take A Deep Breath

Taking very deep breaths usually has an amazing calming effect when you are very anxious. It is especially helpful when the panic attack manifests itself by ridding you of breath, so that you are constantly gasping for breath. As you breathe in and out deeply, close your eyes and empty your mind of every thought. Doing this for five minutes will go a long way in helping you calm down and gain more control of your body.

Create the worst case scenario

Sometimes, your worst fears are fuelled by your imagination. They may seem very real and plausible when you are anxious, but when you look back afterwards, you realize that they are nothing short of ridiculous. You have to train your brain how to challenge your worst fears when you are feeling anxious. Ask yourself what the worst thing that could happen to you is. When you critically analyze your fears and see how impractical they are, then you will have an easier time battling anxiety.

Talk to someone

It is often said that a problem shared is a problem half solved, and the saying holds even for anxiety. When you feel your anxiety getting the best of you, be quick to call or talk to someone you trust. Sometimes, saying your fears out loud has a way of minimizing them, and you suddenly start feeling that you can actually overcome them.

Anxiety can be dreadful. The good news, however, is that there are things you can easily do to calm yourself down when panic attacks. Do not let anxiety get the best of you- fight it with all your might and it will lose its grip on you.

Chapter 16
How To Calm Yourself Down in Stressful Situations

When faced by a stressful situation what can we do? Ideas below, are practical and can be used in emergencies or when you realize that you have been carrying a low level of stress for awhile. We'll explore several ways that are easy and practical.

First, what does the body do when it is stressed and how can I identify low-level stress? We need to be aware of how the body responds to stress, because if we can catch it before it 'takes us over,' it is much easier to 'tame.'

PHYSIOLOGICAL SIGNS OF STRESS

When we find ourselves in a stressful situation we often find that we:

1. Begin to breathe more rapidly. Our body is getting the 'fight and flight' response ready so that we can run of the fight.

2. Find our heart pumps faster to give us more blood for our fight or flight; we might get heart palpitations, chest pains or begin to feel flushed. Our heart is giving all it has to help us in our flight.

3. Our blood pressure increases to pump more blood into our body so that we can run or fight. We might get a headache or pressure in our head.

4. Feel tight, anxious, nervous and irritable. The hormone Cortisol begins to rush through our body getting us ready for flight or flight. This pushes all of to the organs and cells to 'get ready.'

So are we going to suffer early aging and illness, which is what long-term stress can do to us? No! We can do something about it. Using tools and techniques, we can turn stress into transformation.

Blow are some ideas to help in 'transforming stress.' Use them often, write them on a stickie note and keep them with you until they become a habit. They say it takes 28 days to make a new habit.

HOW TO CALM YOURSELF DOWN AFTER A STRESSFUL SITUATION.

1 Take deep three breaths and let them out slowly.

2 Now squeeze your hands and feet and release the squeeze slowly.

3 Put the corners of your lips up and do #1 again.

4 Take a walk or exercise. Nature helps to cut stress as do animals and birds. So go ahead and hug your cat or dog they will love it and it can seriously cut stress.

5 Take an Epsom salt or sea salt bath, put some lavender oil in and relax with deep breathing.

6 Whistles, sing, or listen to your favorite soothing music...music can change your mood almost instantly.

7 Call a friend chat about something fun or meet them for tea.

8 Give thanks for ten things in your life.

9 Carry soothing lavender and dab it on your wrists, it is very soothing.

10 Carry soothing lavender and dab it on your wrists, it is very soothing.

Stress can make our life feel so difficult, as if its so much of a struggle, but using these tools can make a significant change to your life if your use them regularly and correctly.

Chapter 17
How to Use the 80/20 Principle to Reduce Stress

The 80/20 rule popularly known as the Pareto Principle was born by an Italian, Vifredo Pareto, after observing that approximately 20% of the people living in Italy owned an astonishing 80% of wealth. It reflected a simple symmetry of inequality then, and the principle gradually spread to other areas of life, particularly stress relief. According to Pareto, the majority of any output comes from the minority of any input.

From a wellness perspective 80% of your health problems will come from 20% of the lifestyle choices you make. Smoking for example, is a small thing that causes many people several health problems. When it comes to stress something that seems trivial would be enough to trigger major problems in some people. Someone might say something about your appearance thinking it's a joke but if you take it to heart, chances are that it will weigh down on your mind. To deal with the negative thoughts you will probably run to the pub for a drink but end up spending money that was meant for your bills. Later you might have to lie and the domino effect of stress continues. Depression easily steals 80% of one's quality of life and most often, we fail to realize that its root cause is not what people say but low self-esteem. Simply working on your confidence would in this case be the 20% you need to do to avoid stress.

In today's society, people with depression or ADHD quickly turn to drugs in a bid to manage the situation but if you were to follow the 80/20 principle, that is a drastic turn. Attention deficit problems, stress and depression are usually as a result of lifestyle choices so the simple solution would be making changes the foods you eat, how you work out and improve your outlook on life.

Anyone can use Pareto's principle to reduce stress especially during this festive season when there are countless matters to attend to. Try making two columns of things that brings you stress and those that bring you joy. If for example you find that shopping causes you a great deal of anxiety, have someone else do it for you so you can focus on activities that bring happiness. Trying to impress others is one of the reasons why many people feel dejected, rejected and unwanted. In line with Pareto's principle you should protect the 80% that encompasses happiness and wellbeing by invoking positive thoughts and embracing simple solutions to seemingly big problems.

Bonus Chapter

General principles of hygiene

The following section gathers principles and natural laws regarding your general health practices. These principles of life hygiene, alone, **could** be the answer to many contemporary diseases. This chapter is written in a rather strange tone, this is deliberately intended.

The purpose of this chapter is to make you aware that your daily habits play a very important role in your health.

Choosing good doctors:

See doctors who respect the laws of nature. When necessary, they will treat you with alternative medicines, which are in harmony with nature. These doctors have learned to analyze the messages your body sends you through its pain signals.

These doctors do not try to conceal your pain and your diseases with artificial substances created by man, which lead you to illness. They know that the illness and pain are nothing but messages, sent by your body, to help you bring order and balance to your life.

They treat you by searching for the causes of your imbalances through dialogue, through the examination of your body, and eventually though scientific analyses such as blood samples or X-rays, so that you can overcome them with their help.

To alleviate your pain, they primarily use plants or tools, which put your organs, your sinews, your nerves, your muscles and your bones back in place, and they work on the balance of your body's energy.

Stay away from doctors who try to conceal your pains and the symptoms of your imbalances, without ever curing you of the causes of your diseases. In order to do that, they always make you use more artificial substances and narcotics created by man.

These only poison you more and more, they aggravate your diseases or cause new ones, and they lead you, irreversibly, to a premature death, sometimes causing great pain.

Microbes and bacteria are not your enemies, but your friends if your body is healthy. They exist to clean your body and strengthen your immune system. You permanently have about one and a half kilograms of microbes and bacteria in your body, which exist in your blood, your lungs and your digestive tract in order to strengthen your immune system and improve your health.

A good doctor does not try to kill your body's bacteria and microbes through antibacterial or antimicrobial preparations, but rather to improve the general condition of your body so as to help the existing microbes and bacteria do their job of cleaning and defending, and thus protect you from diseases. Bad doctors do the opposite.

It is almost like they try in vain to eliminate mosquitoes and microbes from swamps, whereas they exist there precisely to clean them up. If a swamp can sometimes be a nuisance, it is enough to clean it up and to dry out the soil by draining the water for the mosquitoes and microbes to disappear on their own, once the swamp has disappeared and the ground has been cleaned up.

The same applies to the human body. Let the microbes and the bacteria continue to do their good work inside your body, and as for you, just cleanse it by respecting the principles of a healthy lifestyle. However, consider that what you read here does not tell you that you must stay away from all doctors.

Medicine has evolved a lot over the centuries. There are very good doctors and it is up to you to find them. A good doctor, if he has to use approved drugs, will rely on hospitals and laboratories in order to investigate the causes of your illnesses and establish his diagnosis with the aim of cleansing your body.

Nutrition:

Over millennia, nature has been constantly improving circulation and strengthening man's immune system. Today, illnesses are not caused by germs, but by unhealthy living habits.

Purifying your body with healthy lifestyle habits will allow you to naturally drive away potential bad germs, viruses and bacteria from your body.

To season your food, you should refrain from using any artificial substance made by man in favor of aromatic herbs and natural spices that come from plants.

Stay away from artificial substances, which are man-made, in your food. These are supposedly preserving your food, improving its texture, adding color or changing its taste. They upset the harmony and the balance of your body.

Stay away from all man-made industrial foods as well and cook your own meals. Processed foods are not only filled with artificial substances, but they are also adulterated and devoid of the essential nutrients and naturally occurring trace elements.

As you have already seen, in order to maintain the elliptical stability of your body, you must refrain from trying to cure yourself with any synthetic drug created by man, or from changing your food, except when it is prescribed to you by a competent doctor. But you must also refrain from any substance that could alter or modify your state of consciousness.

Thus, you must refrain from synthetic substances such as heroin, derived from the poppy plant, or cocaine, derived from the Kola tree. These synthesized or refined plants alter, stimulate or numb your natural sense perceptions.

Originally, all narcotics come from plants, which exist to be used with wisdom, only in the art of medicine, or for the decoration of your environment.

You should also understand that each time you pierce your skin or your organs, such as your tongue or your teeth, to hook something to it or mix up different metals and other materials, you are not respecting your body. Your body is a miracle in itself.

The same applies when you change the texture of your skin, or of your teeth, by incorporating foreign substances, such as ink, quicksilver or lead. By piercing or changing your skin harmony in particular, and that of your body in general, without a medical prescription, you are not respecting your body.

If you have already done such things then you should definitely break away from them and restore your health.

You should not smoke any plant. Tobacco, heroin and cannabis are made to treat contusions and certain diseases.

No plant exists to be smoked. They exist to please the eye, to be used for food or, as already mentioned, to be used with wisdom, in the art of medicine or for the decoration of your environment.

You should limit your tea and coffee consumption to a maximum of 3 cups a day. Beyond this quantity, the theine and caffeine molecules contained in these hot drinks affect synaptic efficacy and shorten your life. Meanwhile and manifestly, your memory, your capacity for analysis and synthesis start to function less effectively.

Also, refrain completely from the industrial cold drinks people have called *sodas* since the 20th century. The artificial additives, such as the sweeteners we find in these drinks, also affect your synaptic efficacy, kill your brain cells and create organic disorders. This will cause diseases, such as the one you know as Alzheimer's disease, and bring about the shortening of your life.

Various fruits and oilseeds, freshly picked, ripe and promptly transported from close to where you live, should be staple foods in your diet. According to your appetite, after washing and peeling them, eat them to the exclusion of other foods, during breakfast. You can also eat them approximately 30 minutes before lunch or dinner, and also between meals.

Feed yourself with the color and the smell of the fruit. In the fruit, feel the life that arouses your taste buds and stimulates your digestive system, as the food enters the depths of your body.

To benefit from this beautiful harmony, when you eat a fruit or a walnut, chew slowly until the fruit becomes juice in your mouth.

In the same way, do not hesitate, if you feel the need, to eat oilseeds between meals, such as walnuts, hazelnuts or cashews, chewing them slowly. This kind of dry fruit turns into vegetable milk in your mouth and they give your body trace elements that are very useful in maintaining your good health.

By doing so, you will notice that, gradually, you will feel less urge for large meals with baked and cooked foods, which require long preparations.

At midday and in the evening, eat as many mixed vegetables as you wish, favoring those you can eat raw. Do not eat them without peeling and washing them thoroughly with running water.

When you are peeling vegetables, including those that grow in the soil such as carrots or potatoes, as well as garlic, onions or mushrooms, do not worry about killing a microscopic living being such as bacteria or microbes, which are conceived so as to be protected from human hands and to live in harmony with man when he peels his vegetables.

Even if you have a high level of hygiene, remember, you have in you, and on you, billions of infinitely small beings of the animal world, such as bacteria and microbes, which contribute to the balance of your skin, of all your organs and particularly of your whole digestive tract.

Rice, wheat and all naturally self-reproducing cereals are the gold grains of your diet.

They are perfectly suited for feeding man if they are not rendered sterile by genetic manipulations. Legumes such as beans, peas, lentils are also necessary on a daily basis, in moderation, complementing your other foods, for building or regenerating your cells, especially your muscles and the balance of your blood.

You must consume these cereals and legumes moderately every day, ideally at midday rather than in the evening, because they contain the elements necessary for building or regenerating your cells, but they take more time to digest than fruits and vegetables.

Between meals, eat 8 or 10 oilseeds such as walnuts, almonds or hazelnuts, but do it by chewing slowly, up to the point of feeling the vegetable milk being released.

Do not drink non-dairy milks or soy milk manufactured in factories, because industrial vegetable-based milk contains virtually no vitamins and natural micronutrients.

In the same way as for the fruits in the morning, whether you eat a raw or a cooked vegetable, a grain or a legume, feed yourself with the color and with the smell of every piece of food you put in your mouth.

When you eat, eat it slowly, with respect, gratitude and appreciation for this living food.

Your body needs to absorb 2 to 3 liters of water a day. Above all, you will get this water from your daily fruit, legumes, raw vegetables and sprouted grain diet.

You will supplement your water needs by additionally drinking, every day between meals (*and never during meals*), 1 to 2 liters of water a day.

Do not drink at all, or drink little, water during your meals so as not to drown or destroy your food's nutrients. By respecting these simple common sense rules, you will enjoy excellent health.

Fasting and Rest:

Today, a very large number of studies highlight the incredible therapeutic and purifying virtues of fasting:

Weight loss, improvement of certain chronic illnesses, improvement of cognitive faculties, cleansing of the digestive system and overall purging for our body, etcetera.

The author assumes that we eat too much and that fasting allows the body to rest and purify itself. The body is then cleansed of old cells, fat, waste and toxins that clutter it.

Fasting has nothing to do with anorexia, which is a disease. It is not dangerous, it is accessible to everyone (except in a few pathological cases), because we have reserves to maintain us without problem for several days.

Several types of fasts exist:
- Water fasting
- Dry fasting
- Intermittent fasting

We invite you to learn all about these types of fasts.

But this is more than just about food, this is a complete philosophy of life. It's about resting from all points of view: media, technology, music.

Why not reduce the amount of time you spend on your phone - the time you spend watching negative news, listening to music for too long at high volume?

All of this is over-stimulating your body.

Although the chapter you have just read is written in a somewhat imperative tone, it is intended to give you some ideas to get you thinking.

The goal is to show you that healthy living plays a very important role in your overall health.

Healthy living is what allows you to accompany healing, and also to prevent the appearance of diseases in the future.

Final Words

Thank you!

Congratulations, you have now reached the end of this book.

You have understood that it is important to take care of yourself and of your body.

Your health should be your top priority.

Because in reality: **Is there anything more precious for human beings than health**?

As always, we advise you to consult your doctor before taking any action. This book is only a collection of pieces of advice that have proven their reliability, but do not forget that, like any other book, it does not replace a quality diagnosis from a qualified physician.

Your Gift: Free eBook about Alkaline Foods

To thank you for having read this book, we offer you a digital book in PDF format that you can read at home!

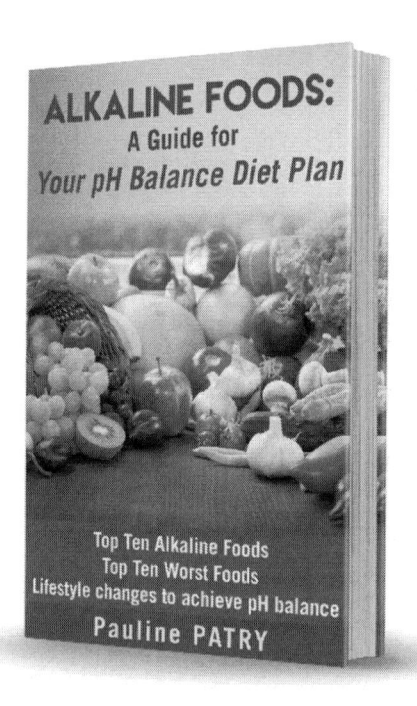

This ebook is about the acid-based equilibrium of your body. You will learn how to regulate this equilibrium. What foods to avoid and what foods to choose.

For a free sample of the book, you can visit this web link:

https://katvio.com/book

You can also Scan the following QR code with your smartphone, it will open the link automatically:

Your Feedback on this eBook

If you think that this book can help other people in distress, take time to share a positive opinion.

If you are not pleased with this book, you can contact the author of this book to share your comments. We are very serious about continuously improving this book. Therefore, if you have a feedback or an improvement to submit, you can directly contact the author using this web link:

https://katvio.com/feedback

Besides, if you think that this book can help other persons, then the best way to let people know is by putting a positive review on the website where you bought the book.

May you be in excellent health!

Pauline PATRY

Printed in Great Britain
by Amazon